Hushed Up Cancer Cures

This publication is part of a Health Series of publications Vol. 7

Copyright © 2017

Prem Chhatwani
Pjan International, Inc.

ALL RIGHTS RESERVED

Disclaimer: This book is not intended as a substitute for the medical advice of your personal medical doctor. The reader should consult a physician before considering any alternate therapies, including chelation, weight loss, cancer and diabetic alternate treatments requiring regular monitoring and diagnosis.

The author and publisher have made every effort to ensure that the information in this book was correct at press time. This book is a simplified version of various treatments and ideas including author's personal experiences and results. Reader may have different experiences and results and hence should be watchful when proceeding with these treatments and procedures.

The author and publisher do not assume and hereby disclaim any liability to any party for any loss, damage, or disruption caused by errors or omissions, whether such errors and omissions result from negligence, accident, or any other cause.

Table of Contents

DEDICATION

I would like to dedicate this book to my Mom and several other people in my family who have been very precious to me at all times.

My dear Mom died at an early age of 55 due to Breast Cancer. That's 20 years ahead of the average life expectancy of American women.

My dear Father who was a great teacher and who taught me great lessons to be kind and be of service to others. He passed away at age of 70 due to Asthma.

My elder sister who cared and loved me since I was growing up. She passed away due to renal failure at an age of 69.

Finally my elder brother who is a great inspiration to me and though is currently undergoing several health issues including Kidney Dialysis, is always upbeat and willing to extend his help to everyone.

Introduction

It is May 24th, 1968 almost 5:00 AM. My Mom is fighting for her last breath. We all in the family including my Dad were around her bed watching her fighting to breath and live. She was on her way to heaven.

Finally she passed away at 5:58 AM at an early age of 55+. She died of Breast cancer diagnosed 5 years earlier. She took radiation treatments however then her doctor gave her 5 years at most. That is what exactly happened!

After watching my Mom die of cancer, I took an oath I will pursue Alternate therapies and help myself and my family and friends.

It is 2017 now and I am 78+ years old and I have taken care of myself and in return published few books on Amazon kindle to help others, if I could.

My family history and genes are real bad. My Dad had Asthma for years and died in 1978 at age of 70 years.

My sister died at age of 69 with renal failure (kidney failure). I was in the same room with her until her last breath.

My brother is of age 82 and had diabetes for several years and had heart bye pass and now his kidneys have failed and is on dialysis, twice / week.

With family history like that I have done all I could to avoid all such problems, so far!

I have no heart issues, B.P., diabetes or any life threatening diseases.

I take good care and follow alternate therapies.

Read my Kindle books on Amazon. Nothing to brag about. Here is the link:

Ok let us talk about Cancer and alternate treatments here in USA.

Did you know that MD Anderson Hospital, in Houston Texas, is one of the leading Cancer hospitals in the world? You see, a handful of doctors — with the support of the hospital's director have decided to buck chemo, radiation, and surgery for their cancer patients.

The same thing is happening at institutions like Baylor... Johns Hopkins... and UCLA.

Surveys by *The Los Angeles Times* and the McGill Cancer Center in Montreal, Canada reveal that **75 percent to 91 percent of oncologists would refuse**

Chemotherapy if they had cancer. They know that it is extremely toxic and not very effective.

According to Dr. Devra Lee Davis, M.P.H., Ph.D., founding director of the world's first Center for Environmental Oncology, "Mammography is one of the most oversold and understudied technologies in medical history.

To continue to assert that mammography will save lives flies in the face of huge numbers of studies on the topic."

Mammograms can actually *increase* a woman's risk of developing breast cancer by as much as *3 percent per*

year by irradiating the breast cells and triggering breast cancer.

Cancer accounts for nearly 1 of every 4 deaths!

And according to the American Cancer Society there will be an estimated 1,665,540 new cancer cases diagnosed and 585,720 cancer deaths in the U.S. this year alone.

Dr. Janet Funk and her team at the University of Arizona are testing this theory by starting to examine bone effects of turmeric in breast cancer. Also   Thaddeus Pace, assistant professor in the UA College of Nursing, is conducting a small pilot study to examine the ability of turmeric to reduce fatigue in women undergoing chemotherapy and radiation treatment for breast cancer.

2. Ozone Therapy

The Oxygen Therapy that Saved Ronald Reagans Life.

In 1985, President Ronald Reagan was scheduled to attend the G7 economic summit in the town of Bonn, Germany. The media created a huge firestorm when Reagan added a visit to a German war memorial cemetery at Bitburg to his schedule.
But what no one knew at the time was that Reagan had another, secret appointment…
You see, Reagan had colon cancer.
I know what you're thinking. "Wait a minute… colon cancer kills fast. But Reagan didn't die of colon cancer. He lived to age of 93 even though he had Alzheimer's. You're right. Colon cancer didn't kill Ronald Reagan.
He beat it.

But not with cancer surgeries and chemotherapy that were standard at the time.

Oh, he had those… Reagan's medical history reveals that he had colon cancer surgery in the U.S. in 1985.

Dr. Oller performed the surgery, and Reagan's doctor, John E. Hutton, participated in the operation.

Yet in 1985, Reagan still visited Dr. Hans Nieper.

According to reports there are no official records of his visit, and no reports on what he was treated for.

But in 1987, Dr. Neiper, who was famous for curing patients of cancer using a special, natural therapy that didn't require surgery, and that saved 50% of "terminal" patients, was interviewed by Videographer Jeff Harsh.

Dr. Nieper talked about his colon cancer work. He simply said "President Reagan is a very nice man."

In 1982, President Ronald Reagan declared April "Cancer Control Month."

He issued Proclamation 4919, and wrote "Research has demonstrated that lifestyle and environment play a crucial role in the development of cancer. We have developed greater understanding of the effects of exposure to carcinogens and have also learned the importance of diet and nutrition as factors in the development and prevention of cancer."

In the same year, 1982, Reagan also fired the entire U.S. Cancer Advisory Board.

Reagan had been saved by a therapy that is not FDA approved for any use, yet over 8,000 MDs and licensed health practitioners in Germany use it in their practices.

What is this radical therapy that attacked Ronald Reagan's cancer so effectively?

Ozone therapy.

Useful Links

1) American Academy of Ozone Therapies:
   http://www.aaot.us

2) Here is a fairly comprehensive directory of ozone therapy doctors and clinics:
   http://www.o3medicalozone.com/ozone-clinics

The Amazing Oxygen Cure

Hyperbaric Oxygen Therapy (HBOT)

HBOT is the latest oxygen therapy that has been shown very effective for treatment of

- Autoimmune diseases;
- Multiple sclerosis;
- Cerebral palsy;
- Migraine headaches;
- Diabetes;
- And even cancer!

  Listen to "Introduction to Hyperbaric Oxygen Therapy"

  https://youtu.be/Zmzf-giAwVg

The therapy itself is actually quite simple. You simply lie down in a pressurized enclosure called a hyperbaric chamber, and inhale 100% oxygen, which first fills the red blood cells in the bloodstream, then continues to flow into the bloodstream and is absorbed directly into the plasma (one of the components of blood).

The increased atmospheric pressure facilitates oxygen absorption. The dissolved oxygen in the plasma is more readily available for use by the cells in the body.

HBOT is a process that floods the body with oxygen so that it may more readily heal itself. And when you deliver pressurized oxygen to your body in this way, it's absorbed into your blood and in your tissues in massive quantities. So blood and plasma is saturated with oxygen delivered to all organs.

These huge doses of oxygen... **Suffocate deadly diseases.** Cancer cells simply cannot survive in oxygen rich blood. Many other diseases cannot survive in oxygen rich environment. Flooding your body with oxygen brings the healing.

- Helps regenerate blood vessels, tissues and nerves. Highly beneficial for people suffering from brain diseases, Alzheimer's, depression and so on.
- HBOT has been commonly used by athletes, NFL players to heal faster from multiple concussions suffered during the games.
- Ideal for people affected by Cluster headaches.
- Increase the power of your immune system and healing power by releasing your own stem cells.
- Helps wipe out inflammation in body, the cause of heart diseases, Cancer and Stress.
  There are now 18 specific conditions that are approved by the FDA for hyperbaric oxygen treatments and many more that are not ("off label conditions") require further research for FDA approval.

FDA approved conditions for treatment with HBOT.

- Air or Gas Embolism

- Exceptional Blood Loss/Anemia

- Carbon Monoxide and Smoke Inhalation Carbon Monoxide Poisoning complicated By Cyanide Poisoning

- Crush Injury

- Decompression Sickness (The Bends)

- Clostridal Myositis and Myonecrosis/Gas Gangrene

- Necrotizing Soft Tissue Infections

- Intracranial Abscess

- Complications Of Radiation Therapy/Radiation Tissue Damage

- Osteomyelitis

- Skin Grafts and Flaps

- Thermal Burns

- Arterial Insufficiencies

- Central Retinal Artery Occlusions

- Non-healing Wounds

- Acute Mountain Sickness

- Idiopathic Sudden Sensorineural Hearing Loss

Some of the "OFF Label" conditions treated with HBOT with documented positive results.

- Traumatic Brain Injury

- □Stroke

- Cerebral Palsy

- Closed Head Injury

- Aids

- Chronic Fatigue Syndrome
- Arthritis
- Limb/Digit
- Reattachment Surgery Recovery
- Tuberculosis
- Hansen's Disease
- Myocardial Infarction
- RSD
- □Conditioning Therapy
- Autism
- Multiple Sclerosis
- Near Drowning
- □Macular Degeneration
- Cancer
- Amputation Recovery
- Spider/Snake Bite
- Epstein Barr
- Plastic Surgery Recovery
- Staph Infection
- Chemotherapy Recovery
- Bells Palsy
- Dementia
- Migraine/Headaches

- Lyme Disease

- Parkinson's Disease

- Coma

Who Cannot Have HBOT?
There are a few conditions in which some may not be able to undergo HBOT. If the patient has certain types of lung damage, hyperbaric oxygen therapy may not be a suitable treatment. Certain medications will also preclude some from hyperbaric oxygen treatment.
☐Diabetics are required to take a blood test before each hyperbaric treatment. If the blood sugar level is too low, the patient will not be permitted to undergo treatment until the level is raised. These conditions are for the overall wellness of the patient.

You can also visit Oxygen Healing Therapies: http://www.oxygenhealingtherapies.com

Directory of Hyperbaric Oxygen Therapy Treatment Centers:

Click on this link below to find a center near you.

http://www.hyperbariclink.com/treatment-centers/treatment-centers.aspx#.VuR3gvkrKM8

Also check on the above site the links on the top tool bar. Very valuable information.

"About Hyperbaric Treatment" and "Directories"

Hyperbaric oxygen is serious medicine that should always be prescribed by a physician. Treatments should always be supervised by a qualified

Hyperbaric specialist physician (MD or DO) assisted by a certified hyperbaric technician (CHT).

HBOT Chambers

There are two basic types of hyperbaric chambers:

- Monoplace chambers are filled with 100% oxygen during treatment and hold one patient. Patients recline during treatment. Most modern monoplace chambers have clear acrylic walls so medical personnel can monitor the patient.

- Multiplace chambers can treat more than one patient at a time and patients can be accompanied by healthcare professionals.

- In multiplace chambers the pressurized atmosphere is a standard mix of gases, and patients receive 100% oxygen through a mask or hood.

Each type of chamber has particular benefits for specific medical problems. Some treatment centers have both monoplace and multiplace chambers.

Side Effects

No effective medical treatment comes without the risk of some adverse reactions. The rates of complication for hyperbaric oxygen therapy are very low. Potentially serious side effects include trauma to the middle ear, the eye (progressive myopia or cataracts), the lungs (pulmonary edema), and the brain (seizure), as well as claustrophobia. The Undersea and Hyperbaric Medical Society provides an informative page on side effects.

Here is link from one of the manufacturer of HBOT equipment showing models for home use. (For informational purposes only. We have no association with this or any other manufacturer).

http://www.newtownehyperbarics.com/ourchambers/class4.html

Note: In USA a prescription is required from a qualified medical professional for human medical use of such devices.

Cost and Reimbursement for Hyperbaric Oxygen Therapy

Fees for hyperbaric oxygen therapy can range from around $200 per treatment in independent clinics to over $1,000 in hospitals, depending on the type of treatment center, physician consultation fees, and other factors. Emergency hyperbaric treatment for acute conditions such as central retinal artery occlusion or necrotizing fasciitis may cost more than routine treatment of a chronic wound at an outpatient clinic.

Fortunately, Medicare, Medicaid, and private insurers generally reimburse for the treatment of approved indications and occasionally reimburse for the treatment of off-label or alternative indications.

Reimbursement rates and criteria may vary widely by insurance carrier, type of treatment center, and by state or region.

Hyperbaric treatment for decompression sickness as a result of a scuba diving accident are generally not covered by standard health insurance plans, but the Diver's Alert Network (DAN), a leading scuba diving safety organization, provides a comprehensive diving insurance program that covers hyperbaric treatment.

I came across this website by Dr. Harch located in New Orleans area. It may be worth reviewing.
http://www.hbot.com/

Here is the basic information from Dr. Harch's website.

If you are interested in being a patient of Dr. Harch, he does telephone interviews with patients & families, in person medical consultations in the New Orleans area, orders SPECT brain imaging through West Jefferson Medical Center, and administers hyperbaric oxygen treatment to patients with neurological and non-neurological indications. "Hyperbaric Oxygen Therapy is simply a viable treatment for wounds in the body in any location and of any duration."

For patients who cannot afford transportation to New Orleans for a consultation/evaluation we have a Christian organization who may fly you here pro bono if you are financially disadvantaged.

For inquiries on consultations or treatment contact:

Dr. Paul G. Harch or Juliette Lucarini RN
Harch HBOT at Family Physicians' Center
5216 Lapalco Blvd
Marrero, LA 70072

(504)309-4948

Listen to DR. Paul Harch at the 8th International Hyperbaric Symposium HBOT 2012 where he explains HBOT treatment of Cancer.

Here is the link:
https://www.youtube.com/watch?v=msmAganFzEY&feature=plcp

You may also visit these sites:

US National Library of Medicine

National Institutes of Health

http://www.ncbi.nlm.nih.gov/pmc/?term=hyperbaric+oxygen+therapy

There are 4791 articles on this site about HBOT Therapy:

Just on Cancer alone there are 1803 articles:

Here is a sampling related to Cancer:
Hyperbaric Oxygen Therapy | Dr. Susan Sprau - UCLA Health System.
https://www.youtube.com/watch?v=cTROb6ZdZjU

It is almost hour and half presentation.

(Watch first 10 minutes at least to get an idea.)

Hyperbaric Oxygen Therapy Chamber (HBOT)

This company is one of the suppliers of this equipment. Just watch this to get the idea.

https://www.youtube.com/watch?v=z739TPEo_hw

4. Proton Therapy

Proton Therapy is much more accurate in targeting tumors compared to radiation therapy commonly used to treat cancer.
Radiation therapy using x-ray beams affect the cancer cells but also damage nearby healthy tissues. That limits the dosage used to target cancer cells.

Proton Therapy is more targeted using positively charged proton particles. The proton beams enter the body with low radiation dose and the dose increases as it enters the target. Thus maximum energy is delivered to tumor. Thus the delivery is more precise and effective.

One of the best Proton Therapy Centers, in US is M D Anderson, Houston Texas. According to their site they also offer Pencil Beam and Intensity Modulated Proton Therapies. Following information appears at their site:

Pencil Beam and Intensity Modulated Proton Therapy

Pencil beam scanning, also known as spot scanning, is a proton therapy technique used to treat complex tumors. Powerful magnets direct thousands of ultra-fine proton beams from multiple directions toward the tumor, creating a protective "U" shape around healthy tissue and avoiding sensitive areas. MD Anderson's Proton Therapy Center currently uses pencil beam scanning to treat cancers of the prostate, brain, base of the skull and eye.

The Proton Therapy Center is also a leader in Intensity Modulated Proton Therapy. This treatment is best used to deliver a potent and precise dose of protons to complex or concave-shaped tumors that may be next to the spinal cord or embedded in the head and neck or skull base, including nasal and sinus cavities, the oral cavity, salivary gland, tongue, tonsils, and larynx.

Watch their video at this link: https://youtu.be/a40fROBtkpI Many top ranking hospitals in USA now offer this Proton Therapy.

Check this video offered by famous Mayo Clinic: https://youtu.be/OTd5dv3VDws

5. Rigvir Therapy--Amazing but True!

It all started in Latvia.

Latvia is located in the continent of Europe, Latvia is a country on the Baltic Sea between Lithuania and Estonia. Its capital is Riga. It covers 62,249 square kilometers of land and 2,340 square kilometers of water, making it the 125th largest nation in the world with a total area of 64,589 square kilometers. ... Latvia shares land borders with 4 countries: Russia, Estonia, Belarus and Lithuania.

What is Rigvir?

Rigvir is a drug containing a live and natural virus (ECHO-7) which has cytolytic and immunomodulating effects. Cytolytic action – finding and destroying malignant cells, applies only to the cancer cells without affecting the normal tissue cells.
The Rigvir Therapy was started and has been perfected at International Virotherapy Center (IVC) in Latvia. It has been tested and proven over more than 2000 cases of Cancer of different types. Since then IVC has trained select centers around the world under their guidelines to offer this treatment.
Please contact them at https://www.virotherapy.eu/ for full details and a treatment center near you.

For US residents the nearest center is in Mexico. For full details of this location please see information provided here.

RIGVIR CANCER VIROTHERAPY CENTER, MEXICO

Name: Hope4Cancer Institute. Website:
http://www.hope4cancer.com/

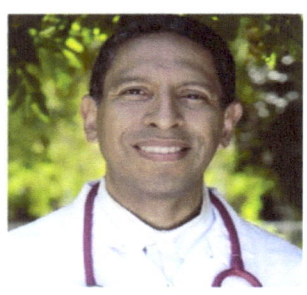

Antonio Jimenez, M.D., Medical Director, Hope4Cancer Institute, Mexico

In my 25 years of treating cancer patients, as well as researching and investigating new cancer treatments, I have never come across a treatment that has a product profile quite like that of Rigvir®. Rigvir® combines excellent efficacy, immune system activation and an unparalleled safety profile. This data is backed by clinical studies conducted over decades that conclusively prove the product's efficacy against a variety of cancers including melanoma, prostate cancer, lung cancer, sarcomas, bladder cancer, uterine cancer and more. Cancer patients owe it to themselves to consider Rigvir® as their treatment of choice."

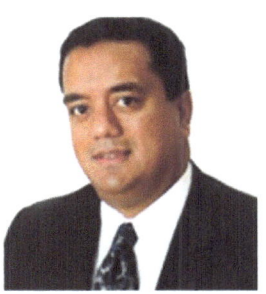

Subrata Chakravarty, Ph.D.   Chief Science Officer, Hope4Cancer® Institute.

Comparing Rigvir® cancer virotherapy to standard chemo-therapy or radiotherapy is similar to comparing the impact of a laser guided Tomahawk missile to that of an atomic bomb. The powerful selective, destructive action, when combined with the avoidance of collateral damage, give Rigvir® an important role in cancer treatment.

Brief message from Hope4Cancer Institute, Mexico

Rigvir® is a registered cancer drug in Latvia that has passed safety and efficacy clinical trials. Developed over the course of last 50 years, Rigvir® represents a paradigm shift in the treatment of cancer. Our partnership with the Latvian Virotherapy Center allows us to bring this affordable treatment to the medicine cabinets of cancer patients around the world.

http://www.hope4cancer.com/

Call us for a free treatment plan approved by Dr. Antonio Jimenez, our Medical Director. Our patient coordinator will be happy to answer your questions and fully discuss your treatment.

Or simply fill out the form on our website. We will respond within the next 48 hours!

Tel. 1-888-544-5993 (Toll Free USA)
    +1-619-669-6511 (USA Based International Number)

Fax. (619) 956-7071

USA Mailing Address:

13910 Lyons Valley Rd., Suite L
Jamul, CA 91935 USA

Mexico Location: Baja California, Mexico
Read Patient Stories here:

**http://www.hope4cancer.com/information/category/pat
ient-stories**

---

6. Dr. Johanna Budwig's Recipe

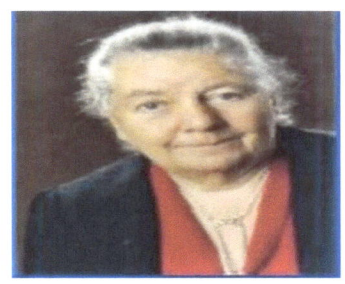

The Budwig Center teaches the **Budwig diet** founded by German biochemist **DR Johanna Budwig**. The Budwig Diet has been successfully helping people with Cancer, Arthritis, Asthma, Fibromyalgia, Diabetes, Blood Pressure, Multiple sclerosis, Heart Disease, Psoriasis, Eczema, Acne and other illnesses and conditions.

Here is the actual information from their site:

To make the Budwig Muesli, blend 2 Tablespoons of organic flaxseed oil (FO) with 4 Table spoons of low-fat(less than 2%) Cottage Cheese (CC) with a hand-held immersion
Electric blender for up to a minute. If the mixture is too thick and/or the oil does not disappear you may need to add 2 or 3 Tablespoons of milk (2% organic milk would be the good option). Do not add water or juices when blending FO with CC. The mixture should be like rich whipped cream with no separated oil.

Remember you must mix ONLY the FO and CC and nothing else at first. Always use organic food products when possible.

Next mix in by hand 1 teaspoon of honey (*raw non-pasteurized is recommended*) or 1 teaspoon of organic Maple syrup (even better).

(Optional) For variety you may add other ingredients such as cinnamon, **chopped almonds**, hazelnuts, walnuts, cashews (no peanuts), and pine kernels. For people who find the Budwig Muesli hard to take these added foods will make the mixture more palatable. Some of our patients have even added a pinch of Celtic sea salt and others put in a pinch of cayenne pepper for a change.

Take this sometime in the morning every day or any other time that works for you.

You will be surprised to start seeing benefits in 4-6 weeks. Do not discontinue.

Also since this is a food it should not interfere with your medication but if you are not sure please consult your doctor.

For additional research click on http://www.budwigcenter.com/wp-content/uploads/2017/03/Johanna-Budwig-Center-Guide-Diet-health.pdf

Note: This is a 50 page document so have patience while it loads. Ton of valuable information.

Caution: Above information is not meant to replace the attention or advice of your physicians or other health care professionals.

Dr. Hulda Clark's Protocol

(Be advised this is a summary of Dr. Hulda Clark's 583 pages book.)

She passed away few years ago but she was a legend in her own way.

Who is Dr. Hulda Clarke?

Hulda Regehr Clark began her studies in biology at the University of Saskatchewan, Canada, where she was awarded Bachelor of Arts, Magna Cum Laude, and the Master of Arts, with high honors. After two years of study at McGill University, she attended the university of Minnesota, studying biophysics and cell physiology. She received her Doctorate degree in physiology in 1958. In 1979 she left government funded research and began private consulting on a full time basis. Eleven years later she noticed clues as to the cause of cancer.

Before publishing her books on Cure for Cancers, Dr. Clark set a goal to cure at least 100 cancer patients to test her theory. She passed that mark in December of 1992. The cure has stood the test of time. Her research has proved that all cancers are caused by a certain Parasite, regardless of the type of Cancer. The parasite is human **intestinal fluke**.

 If you kill this parasite, the cancer stops immediately.

Typically this parasite lives in human intestine causing no harm. May be causing only Crohn's disease, IBS and colitis. However if this parasite settles down in liver, it causes cancer! Further, this happens with people who have isopropyl alcohol (IPA) in their bodies.

All cancer patients (100%) have IPA (the solvent) and this intestinal fluke parasite in their liver.

What is intestinal fluke parasite?

The scientific name is " Fasciolopsis buski". Fluke means "flat". These are family of flatworms. The parasite has been known since 1925.

The adult parasite stays stuck to our intestine. If in liver, causing cancer, or in uterus, causing endometriosis, or in thymus, causing Aids, or in

Kidney, causing Hodgkin's disease. In normal healthy people the parasite does not survive.

Flukes and Isopropyl Alcohol: People who have isopropyl Alcohol in their bodies, their liver is not able to kill these parasites and they begin to multiply. From eggs to adult stage these parasites then eat and suck your body fluids. As soon as they are adults a growth factor called *orthophosphotyrosine* appears. These growth factors make cells divide. Now you have a CANCER!

Purge The Parasite, Cure the Cancer:

The good news is when this fluke, the parasite is terminated, in 24 hours all orthophosphotyrosine is gone! Your Malignancy is gone. Your Cancer can not come back. You have won the battle for your life.
Then all we have to do a cleaning and repair job.

So basically:

1. Kill the parasite and all its stages (Eggs and all)

2. Stop letting isopropyl Alcohol into your body

3. Flush out the metals, common toxins and bacteria from your body.

The Solution - The Herbal Parasite Remedies: Just for your information our body is full of worms and all kinds of parasites.   For example:

 * **Eczema is due to round worms**

* **Seizures are caused by a single roundworm called** *Ascaris***, getting into your brain.**

* **Schizophrenia and depression are caused by parasites in the brain.**

* **Asthma is caused by** *Ascaris* **in the lungs**.

* **Diabetes is caused by the pancreatic fluke called** Eurytrema.

* **Migraines are caused by the thread worm,** Strongyloides.

* **Acne is caused by** Leishmania.

* **Much of heart disease is caused by dog heart worm**, Dirofilaria.

And the list goes on!

Getting rid of all these parasites is impossible with clinical medicines. In addition these medicines have side effects like nausea and vomiting.

Now the Good News! There are just three Herbs **if taken together** will kill over 100 types of parasites. No side effects or interference with any drug that you are already on. They are nature's gift to us.

* Black Walnut Hulls from Black Walnut tree.

* Wormwood from Artemisia shrub.

* Common Cloves from the clove tree.

These three herbs must be taken together to kill adult parasites and the eggs which will develop into adults if not killed.

So here is what we need to start:

* One ounce (30 ml) of pale green Black Walnut Hull Tincture Extra Strength. This is enough for three weeks. 2 ounce bottle costs about $13.79.

* One bottle (about 100 capsules) of wormwood (each capsule with 200-300 mg of wormwood). 365 mg 100 caps cost about $13.99.

* One bottle of freshly ground cloves (500 mg, 100 caps cost $8.49).

In addition to these herbs, two additional items, **Ornithine** and **Arginine** will improve this recipe. Parasites produce a great deal of ammonia as their waste product and is set free in our bodies. It is toxic causing insomnia by night and anxiety by day.

By taking **Ornithine** at bedtime, one would sleep better. **Arginine** should be taken in the morning as it gives alertness and energy.

Ornithine 500mg, 100 caps cost about $14.29.

Arginine 500mg, 100 caps cost about 11.79

Parasite Killing Program.

1. Black Walnut Hull Tincture Extra Strength: (Source: New Action Products, Self-health resource center. See at the end contact information)

Day 1: Take one drop and put it in a 1/2 cup of water and sip it on empty stomach before meals.

Day2. Take two drops same way

Day3. Take 3 drops same as above

Day4. Take 4 drops as above.

Day5. Take 5 drops.

Day6. Take 2 tsp. all together in 1/2 cup of water.

Sip it slowly. Don't gulp it. Add sweetening or fruit sauce and get it down within 15 minutes. (If you are over 150 pounds use 2-1/2 tsp or if over 200 pounds take 3 tsp)

You can use lukewarm water to evaporate some of the alcohol in the tincture.

Then on, 2 tsp. once a week for a year.

Take 500mg of niacinamide (from Self Health Resource Center, Spectrum Chemical Co.) to counteract effect of alcohol in the tincture. If you feel slight nausea for few minutes, walk in the fresh air or simply rest.

Note for Extremely ill or terminally ill Cancer patients:

Take 2 tsp. of this dose every hour for 5 hours. Follow this the same day or next day with Mop up program. if this gets you out of the hospital bed, repeat this every other day for 2 more weeks, before settling for maintenance program once a week. Include wormwood and clove capsules 10 of each with each treatment.

8. Listen to These Doctors and Their Patients

Al Sears, MD, 11905 Southern Blvd.
Royal Palm Beach, FL 33411

561-784-7852

Al Sears, MD is a medical doctor and one of the nation's first board-certified anti-aging physicians.

As a board-certified clinical nutritionist, strength coach and ACE certified fitness trainer, he enjoys a worldwide readership. Dr. Sears has appeared on more than 50 national radio programs, ABC News, CNN, and ESPN.

Take a look at this controversial lab photo from a new study at the University of South Florida.

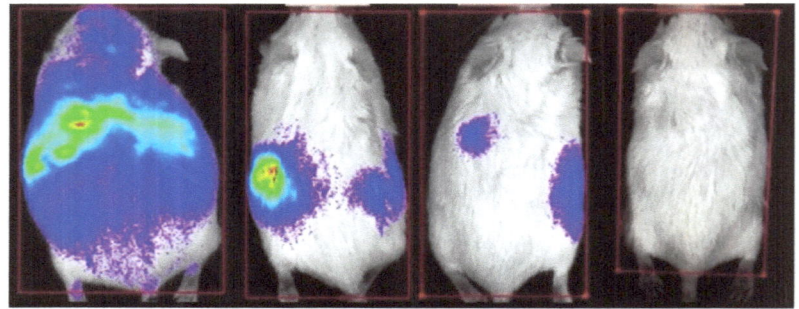

The researchers used "bioluminescence" to mark and illuminate the tumors and where the cancer was spreading. That's where the colors come from.

The first mouse on your left, is your typical cancer patient, treated with chemo and radiation.

It still has all of its tumors and never went into complete remission.

But with this new discovery, the mouse made a complete transformation. The picture on the far right is the same mouse after receiving a very different therapy...

One that includes a protocol, ==Dr. Sears calls *"8th Element."*==

==*In just three weeks, the tumors vanished.*==

All without dangerous side effects, prescription drugs, or invasive surgeries.

According to Dr. Sears one can apply the 8th element protocol from the comfort of your home. Dr. Sears also recommends boosting your immune system. He prefers I V therapies. One of his protocol is "Myer's cocktail".

It is administered by IV and typically contains a potent mix of **magnesium, calcium, vitamin C** and a **B-vitamin complex**. It's specially designed to boost your immune system and restore your energy levels. **Great for recovery from the effects of Chemotherapy.**

*In addition he has now added another powerful ingredient into the Myers' mix — **glutathione**. This is a*

vital protein, antioxidant and detoxifying agent. Three most powerful ingredients are;

- **Glutathione:** This is your body's most potent antioxidant. I've been recommending ways to boost my patients' glutathione levels for years to help them

- Live long and well. It's a critical part of your body's natural mechanism for warding off disease.

- The evidence of glutathione's power is backed up by research and numerous scientific studies. Danish researchers compared people aged 100 to 105 with people aged 60 to 79 — and found the centenarians had much higher levels of glutathione. And those who were most active had the very highest levels. Glutathione increases energy, fights illness, increases mental clarity, reduces body fat, and protects against age-related decline. You can also "cook up" glutathione in your cells if you have three necessary amino acids on board — glycine N-acetyl cysteine (NAC) and glutamic acid (glutamate). One easy way is to supplement with **whey protein**. But be sure to get pure whey from pasture-raised animals, so it's free of toxins and hormones.

- You can get the "reduced form" in a glutathione supplement. This is the only supplement form that's absorbed by your cells.

- **Vitamin C:** This powerful antioxidant is a powerful anti-cancer fighter, especially when given in high dosages. More than 18,000 studies in the PubMed database alone show health benefits of vitamin C. Because humans do not manufacture vitamin C internally, you need to get it through dietary sources or supplements. But the daily intake of 60 mg recommended by mainstream medicine is not enough. Based on my own experience, I recommend 3,000 mg per day if you're in good health and up to 20,000 mg in times of stress or sickness. But taking high dosages of vitamin can upset your stomach, which is why **I recommend IV treatment**.

- **Magnesium:** Modern farming methods have pretty much eradicated magnesium from our soil. But this crucial element balances potassium, sodium and calcium — all of which supports a healthy immune system and prevents the chronic inflammation at the root of all chronic diseases. In fact, getting enough magnesium can lower your risk of dying from any cause. A recent study on 4,203 people found that chances of dying are 10

- times higher for those with the lowest levels of magnesium.

  To supplement with magnesium alone, I recommend getting between 600 mg and 1,000 mg a day. Look for magnesium that is bound to citrate, malate or aspartate. **Take it with vitamin B6.** It will increase the amount of magnesium that ccumulates in your cells.

Stem Cell Therapy

> **Dr. Dipnarine Maharaj, MD**, who is on Dr. Al Sears' Anti-aging dream team and who helped establish the bone Marrow and stem cell transplant programs at the University of Miami...revealed how his stem cell therapy treatment brought long-term survival to 60% of terminal cancer patients by restoring their damaged immune systems!

Disclaimer: I have no relation of any kind with this or any other doctor mentioned in my book here. I am just an information provider providing you all the information as one stop shopping. You judge your best options. There is hope and these doctors are doing something that mainstream doctors do not want to talk about.

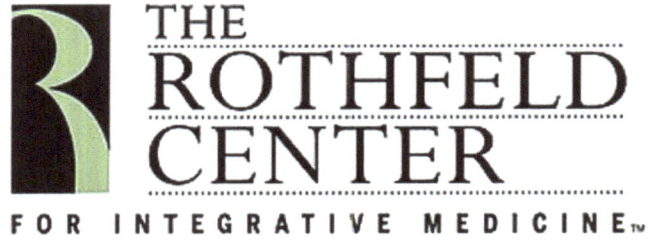

The Rothfeld Center & Apothecary
465 Waverley Oaks Road, Suite 201
Waltham, MA 02452

Phone: 781.736.1901

http://www.rothfeldcenter.com

Founded by Glenn S. Rothfeld MD, The Rothfeld Center offers a comprehensive approach to healthcare rooted in over 35 years' experience in complementary and conventional therapies.

The Rothfeld Center provides a health care setting that combines scientific diagnosis with alternative healing traditions. Dr. Glenn Rothfeld is a fully-licensed MD and acupuncturist whose expertise spans conventional and non-traditional medicine.

Here are the advances in cancer treatments that are offering patients new hope:

Immunotherapies

Typically, when our immune system is faced with a threat — germs or viruses, for instance — it makes antibodies to target and kill the bugs.

Cancer researchers have now created manmade antibodies, called monoclonal antibodies, designed to attach to and kill cancer cells by marking them for destruction by the immune system.

Monoclonal antibodies have been effective in treating a wide range of cancers, including lung cancer, breast cancer and lymphoma.

One of the first of these man-made antibodies, Herceptin, changed the landscape for treatment of HER2-positive breast cancer from one that was "the worst type of breast cancer" to one that nearly always responds to treatment if caught early, says Gordon Mills, professor of medicine and immunology at MD Anderson Cancer Center in Houston.

In the last year, doctors have seen great success with a new type of monoclonal antibody called a checkpoint inhibitor. First approved for treating metastatic melanoma in 2014 and non-small cell lung cancer in 2015 and for metastatic melanoma a few months later, checkpoint inhibitors were used to treat former President Jimmy Carter, who was diagnosed with metastatic melanoma in the fall of 2015; his cancer is now in remission.

Checkpoint inhibitors work by blocking the signal — called a checkpoint — that cancer cells send out telling the immune system not to attack. "The drugs allow the immune system to recognize the tumor," says Svetomir Markovic, an oncologist and hematologist at the Mayo Clinic in Rochester, Minn. Even when patients stop therapy after a few months, the immune system is no longer fooled by the misleading signal. "The early successes of the checkpoint inhibitors have absolutely ignited the scientific community."

Much work lies ahead. The new immunotherapy drugs still only work in about 20 percent of patients overall. But "this advancement of therapeutic strategy where the body's own immune system is the hammer that kills the tumor" has made many oncology practices "literally unrecognizable" from where they were 15 years ago, Markovic says.

Targeted gene therapies

One of the great discoveries in cancer treatment is that cancer tumors have their own genetic footprint. In the last few years, doctors have been able to use that information to test for genetic mutations within an individual's cancer cells and subsequently determine which tumors will be responsive to new medications.

The introduction of these drugs signaled the arrival of a new era particularly in the treatment of leukemia and lymphoma — blood and bone marrow cancers that claim the lives of more than 56,000 people a year.

Before 2001, patients with chronic myeloid leukemia had a life expectancy of 3 to 5 years. Today, many patients who began treatment with one of the first targeted therapy to be approved by the FDA "Gleevec" are still alive 15 years later.

Scientists began searching for other mutations that made the tumors sensitive to new drugs, says Mayo Clinic thoracic surgeon Dennis Wigle.

Several of these new gene-targeted drugs are finally making a difference in lung cancer — by far the nation's deadliest cancer — resulting in "sea change" in how that cancer is treated today, Wigle says. While the drugs don't cure the cancer, in some cases, they can force it into remission, he says. The downside? Many of these drugs have to be taken for a lifetime.

Powerful combinations

For some cancers, using a combination of immunotherapy and targeted medications offers the best chance for success.

The blood cancer multiple myeloma is one of the best examples of this approach, says S. Vincent Rajkumar, a hematologist and oncologist at the Mayo Clinic.

Using medications that cut off a tumor's blood supply, man-made antibodies that target molecules on the surface of cancer cells, medicines that trigger cell death, and bone marrow transplants and Chemotherapy, doctors have drastically increased the prognosis for these patients, from 2 years to a decade or more.

"With the newer therapies, we're turning cancer from a lethal disease into a curable disease," adds Michael atkins, deputy director of Georgetown's Lombardi Center.

Mark Stengler, N.M.D

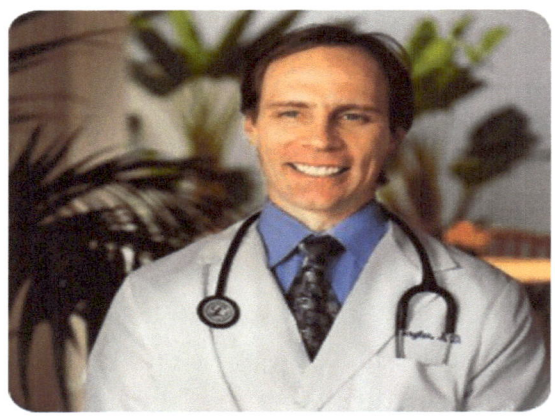

Mark Stengler, N.M.D., is a licensed naturopathic medical doctor and an author. He is considered one of the leaders in the field of integrative medicine, in which the best of holistic and conventional medicine are combined. Dr. Stengler is the author/coauthor of more than thirty books, including several bestsellers. His most recent book is Prescription for Natural Cures, 3rd edition. He has served on a medical advisory committee for the Yale University Complementary Medicine Outcomes Research Project. Dr. Stengler has been interviewed on dozens of television shows on Fox, CBS, NBC, and PBS. He is the author of one of the nation's largest health newsletters, Health Revelations. He maintains a private practice in Encinitas, California. His Web site is www.markstengler.com.

Frank Shallenberger, MD

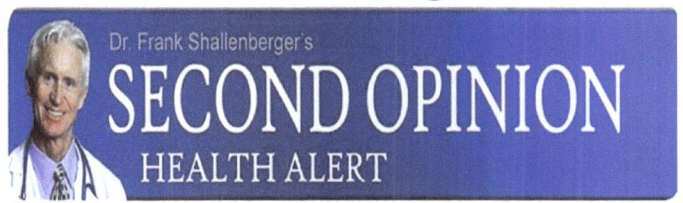

To read all about DR. Shallenberger's credentials please visit

http://www.secondopinionnewsletter.com/Why-Dr-Frank.htm

One simple pill stops breast, prostate, and thyroid cancers

Are you taking iodine? You do if you are my patient. **I recommend iodine to all of my patients because I believe it will prevent breast and prostate cancers.**

Iodine is critical for the formation of thyroid hormones. And thyroid hormones are essential for life. They are the hormones that specifically tell the cells to do what they are supposed to do. So when you're iodine deficient, your cells stop working and things start falling apart. The brain then registers this and sends stimulating signals to the thyroid to produce the hormones the body needs so badly. This causes the thyroid to overwork, and eventually the over stimulation of the thyroid gland can result in the formation of an aggressive thyroid cancer.

The best form of iodine is called Lugol's solution. It was developed way back in 1829 by, you guessed it, Dr. Lugol. It is a mixture of potassium iodide and elemental iodine. You can buy it at Amazon.com in either a liquid or a tablet. The tablet form is the best way to take it. The dose I recommend for all adults is one 12.5 mg tablet per day. But what about testing, you say?

By the way, 12.5 mg is the average amount of iodine that Japanese men and women get in their diets. And the Japanese have lower risks for both prostate and breast cancer. But here's an interesting statistic. When Japanese men and women move to the U.S. and adopt an American diet, which contains only a fraction of the iodine the traditional Japanese diet has, they have the same cancer risks as Americans have.

What every cancer patient must take with chemotherapy

Frank Shallenberger, MD

What they are saying here is that melatonin decreases the toxicity of chemotherapy while at the same time increasing its ability to kill cancer cells.

Clearly the melatonin dramatically improved the efficiency of the chemo drugs and dramatically reduced side effects and improved the quality of life.

The researchers looked at 250 men and women. 104 with lung cancer, 77 had breast cancer, 42 had GI tract cancer, and 27 had head and neck cancers.

They gave some of the patients in each group 20 mg per day of melatonin in addition to their regular chemotherapy. The rest did not get the melatonin supplement. They used the following chemotherapy drugs: cisplatin, etoposide, gemcitabine, doxorubicin, mitoxantrone, paclitaxel, and 5-FU.

Here's what happened.

Specifically, the chemotherapy was effective in killing the tumors in 34% of the patients taking the melatonin compared to only 15% in the non-melatonin group.

The results mean that if you take melatonin along with your chemotherapy, your treatments will be more than twice as effective and you will be more than twice as likely to be alive a year later.

The melatonin also dramatically reduced side effects and improved the quality of life. Listen to the researchers once again. "Moreover, the concomitant administration of melatonin significantly reduced the frequency of thrombocytopenia [platelet destruction], neurotoxicity [nerve damage], cardiotoxicity [heart damage], stomatitis [mouth sores], and asthenia [weakness and poor appetite]. This study indicates that the pineal hormone melatonin may enhance the efficacy of chemotherapy and reduce its toxicity, at least in advanced cancer patients of poor clinical status."

Please get a second opinion from a practitioner who is well versed in natural therapies for cancer. Melatonin may be the single best overall natural anti-cancer therapy.

Dr. Isaac Eliaz

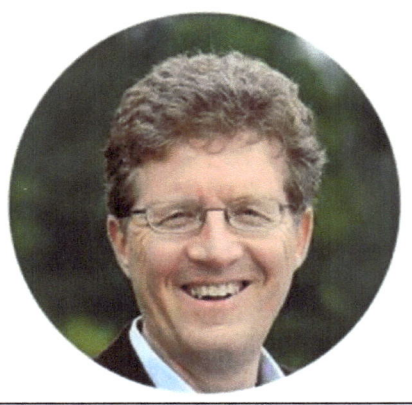

is a renowned integrative medical doctor, licensed acupuncturist, researcher, product formulator and frequent guest lecturer. He has been a pioneer in holistic medicine since the early 1980s, and has published numerous peer-reviewed research papers on several of his key integrative health formulas. He is the founder and medical director of Amitabha Clinic in California, an integrative health center specializing in cancer and chronic conditions. Dr. Eliaz is an expert in using highly strategic, synergistic protocols to address numerous areas of health including metastatic cancer, immunity, digestion, detoxification, diabetes, cardiovascular health and more. His approach integrates modern science with traditional healing wisdom for optimal health and wellness. To download any of Dr. Eliaz's comprehensive wellness guides, click here.

 I spoke recently at Annie Appleseed Project's 10thAnnual Complementary & Alternative Therapies Conference. Annie Appleseed Project has the critical mission of questioning the medical establishment's narrow cancer therapy dogma and offering complementary approaches to help people prevent, treat and survive cancer.

The conference was held in West Palm Beach, from February 25 to 27, and was a lively participatory event with a wide range of topics including developing an anticancer diet and lifestyle, use of anticancer medicinal herbs, and use of medical cannabis.

One of the conference's themes was attacking the underlying factors that contribute to cancer development, growth and metastasis. I spoke about three related subjects: growth factors, inflammation and detoxification. Chronic inflammation is now being recognized as one of the pivotal underpinnings of abnormal cell growth and communication.

Toxins, including heavy metals, pesticides, etc. are another piece of the puzzle, problematic because they tend to spur inflammation and have hormone disrupting effects as well, often stimulating growth promoting estrogens in both men and women.

Botanicals and detoxification fight chronic inflammation

First, there are a number of botanicals and bioactive compounds derived from plants that have been shown to modulate cancer growth and invasion, such as modified citrus pectin, quercetin, turmeric, honokiol, DIM and others. In addition, medicinal mushrooms modulate the immune system, helping it respond better to cancer and other threats.

In my talk I emphasized the importance of addressing chronic inflammation and toxic burden as part of an integrative approach to prevention and treatment.

I recommend modified citrus pectin to address both issues. MCP is known for its ability to bind to heavy metals and other toxins and remove them from the body. MCP also has an affinity for galectin-3, an inflammatory protein that has been shown in numerous studies to be an instigator and driver of cancer progression as well as other major diseases including kidney, liver and cardiovascular disease.

Please visit his website for more information.
http://www.dreliaz.org/

(Note: I have no relation with any doctor. I am just information provider)

Michael Cutler, M.D.

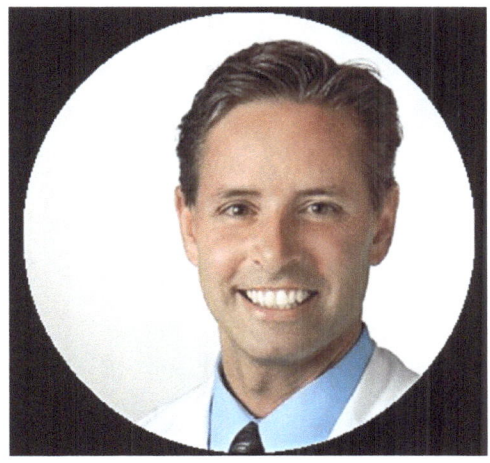

Address: 12285 Scripps Poway Pkwy, Suite #103, Poway, CA 92064.

Tel: 858-208-3676

Website: https://www.drmichaelcutler.com/

According to Dr. Cutler modern medicine is clueless on the importance of insulin.

Now, before you stop reading and say, "Oh, I don't have diabetes," I have some news for you. When you're insulin isn't working right, it's a culprit behind most of the chronic diseases we have today...

- **Heart disease**... (it's not cholesterol)

- **Osteoporosis**... (it's not from lack of calcium)

- **Vision loss**... (it's not because you're getting old)

- **Diabetes**... (it's not just about blood sugar)

- **Alzheimer's**... (Why do you think researchers are starting to call it "type III diabetes?) and most importantly...**Cancer**

How to Build a Cancer-Proof Super-Body!

Did you know insulin is the master control hormone in your body? When it's working right, you can prevent almost every chronic disease we know of, even cancer.

Unfortunately, when insulin is not working right, you have a much *greater* risk for cancer.

Conventional medicine does NOT want you to know the truth about this.

They don't want you to know that when you rejuvenate your insulin function...

Which I can show you how to do easily, without medication. That you can eliminate cancer risk, and the threat of almost every disease we know of.

In helping many patients for over 20 years in clinical and family practice, I've come to realize the importance behind insulin.

Note: Please contact Dr. Cutler for full details if interested. As mentioned before, I have no relationship with any doctor mentioned in this book. So please pursue what you believe in. All the best.

9. Hydrogen Peroxide Protocol

You can't become immune from disease simply by exercising or by being physically fit. Some of the greatest athletes of our time, including 7-time Tour de France champion Lance Armstrong, Olympic ice skating champions Scott Hamilton and Peggy Fleming, and basketball star Magic Johnson, have all been victims of cancer or HIV.

The absolute best way to eradicate disease from your life is by supplying the cells and tissues of your body with its most essential element—and that's oxygen.

Oxygen creates an environment in the body that enables the body to CURE ITSELF of virtually all diseases characterized by viruses, harmful bacteria, toxins, disease microorganisms and pathogens, including but not limited to cancer, AIDS, Alzheimer's and Parkinson's Disease, diabetes, rheumatoid arthritis, multiple sclerosis, heart disease, ulcers, asthma and many other types of diseases, including the flu.

But it's important to remember that sufficient amounts of oxygen need to be supplied at the CELLULAR level. Unless oxygen is delivered to the cells and tissues of the body, it cannot create an environment in the body that is uninhabitable by disease.

One established way to do this is Hyperbaric Oxygen Therapy (HBOT) is described in earlier chapter in this book. HBOT is FDA approved as well.

Additional procedure is the use of **Food Grade Hydrogen Peroxide**.

This therapy moves oxygen atoms from the bloodstream to the cells at a much faster rate than all other means.

This therapy is simple and can be administered at home and is painless. It uses 35% Food Grade H2O2 (Hydrogen Peroxide)

35% Food Grade Hydrogen Peroxide is exactly what is recommended in

The True Power of Hydrogen Peroxide, Miracle Pathway to Wellness by Mary Wright,

One Minute-Cure by Madison Cavanaugh.

Dr. Rowen's ***Second Opinion Newsletter.***

Dr. David G. Williams, ***Hydrogen Peroxide:***

Medical Miracle by William Campbell Douglass II, and

Hydrogen Peroxide & Ozone by Conrad LeBeau.

You simply drink 6-8 ounces of distilled water mixed with few drops of food grade hydrogen peroxide.

The food grade Hydrogen Peroxide is very cost effective, but should be handled carefully and stored in refrigerator.

In "One Minute Cure" by Madison Cavanaugh. She describes on page 74, day by day dosage, using 35% food grade hydrogen peroxide. However 35% grade is bit risky to handle and can cause skin discoloration. I would use small amber color 1oz bottle with dropper. Simply fill the 1 Oz small bottle with 35% food grade H2O2. Use latex gloves for safety. You can buy 35% grade in 8 Oz bottles. Store everything in refrigerator and label everything to avoid accidental misuse!

Here is Amazon link in USA.

http://www.amazon.com/Certified-Hydrogen-Peroxide-Dropper-bottle/dp/B00PBB268M/ref=sr_1_1_s_it?s=hpc&ie=UTF8&qid=1457979291&sr=1-1&keywords=1+OZ+35%25+food+grade+H2O2

Note: This therapy is not for everybody. Seek professional help before using this.

It has only in recent history that the curious relationship between minerals and hydrogen peroxide at the atom level has been explored. It was discovered that without fire, electricity, heat or any device of any kind, there is so much power in combining hydrogen peroxide with certain minerals it could (and has) literally propelled rockets in space. Under a microscope, there is a curious "dance" between minerals and hydrogen peroxide as they interact at the sub-atomic level.

The hydrogen peroxide reacts to the minerals - specifically the second oxygen atom - literally shattering the minerals to their individual atoms - which in turn breaks apart the hydrogen peroxide molecule to release the oxygen. At the sub-atomic level, huge levels of energy are produced and released in this interaction.

Oxygen Therapy with Food Grade Hydrogen Peroxide
https://www.youtube.com/watch?v=N18_YSRDCOQ

It is known that LACK OF OXYGEN reduces mental function, the ability to focus and even to be rational.

Intravenous Hydrogen Peroxide Therapy

The most common method of receiving hydrogen peroxide is through intravenous injection.

Intravenous hydrogen peroxide therapy was first brought to the medical field at the First International Conference of Bio-oxidative Medicine in 1989.

Since then, many people stand behind the supposed power of hydrogen peroxide IV infusions.

Treatments typically last an hour and a half. They can vary in frequency, as some people might request only one treatment and others might want an infusion five days a week. Hydrogen peroxide also has been found to dissolve cholesterol and calcium deposits associated with atherosclerosis. Therefore, it is a good treatment for vascular disorders. This can result in lessening or disappearance of angina, leg pain and transient ischemic attacks to the brain, which cause dizziness. It also can help reverse some of the damage left over by a stroke, if treatment is instituted early enough.

Research in the 1960s at Baylor University showed conclusively that intra-arterial hydrogen peroxide dissolves plaque in large arteries. This makes H2O2 a wonderful complement to EDTA in the treatment of vascular disease, as EDTA has been shown to clear small vessels and create collateral circulation around large vessel blockages. This combination is called "Chelox Therapy."

It also clears the lungs, in cases of emphysema, by producing oxygen bubbles in the alveoli (tiny air sacs in the lungs), literally lifting the mucus deposits up, so they can be coughed out.
Hydrogen peroxide has a remarkable clearing effect on the skin. After only a few intravenous treatments the skin

takes on a translucent clarity usually seen only in children. In addition, hydrogen peroxide benefits asthma, leukemia, multiple sclerosis, degenerative spinal disc disease and high blood pressure. It is particularly effective with asthma, arthritis and back disorders.

If hydrogen peroxide is so effective, why is it not made use of in "modern" medicine? The reason is simple. Hydrogen peroxide cannot be patented. It is present in the ocean, it is present in rainwater, it is present in vegetables, and it is present in every cell of your body right now. It must be classified as a food, because it is part of all fresh food of plant origin. Because it is produced in the human body, it is undeniably safe. Since it is a food and cannot be patented, there is no big profit to be made on it.

There are uncounted hundreds of thousands of lives lost each year from toxicity well-known to the FDA, toxicity which is printed right on the package insert which comes with the drug. Most of these drugs are "chemotherapeutic agents," like AZT and Tamoxifen, designed to treat (not really) terminal conditions. They do not work to cure these conditions, but they do treat the conditions, getting rid of the patient by destroying the immune system — no more disease, but no more patient either.

10. Can Magnetic Therapy Work?

In 1936 Albert Roy Davis was the first scientist who established that the magnet has two distinct North and South poles each having opposite energies. In 1940 he and his research associate Walter C. Rawls, Jr were experimenting with magnets to treat cancer. They found that North Pole energy of a magnet can kill cancer cells.

Since then many researchers have conducted several experiments, according to Journal of National Medical Association, with powerful magnets (3000-4000 Gauss) proving that exposure to north polarity was able to decrease the growth of cancer cells.

Today we know it is proven that magneto therapy is widely used and is effective in treating several diseases. It has been widely used in India, Japan and Russia and now is getting popular in USA.

Several books are available including "Magneto Therapy, Self-Help-Book" by Dr. Bansal, available at www.healingwithmagnets.org in USA.

According to research when a magnet is placed on the skin it exerts a powerful attraction to the iron in our blood. The depth of penetration from the skin depends on the power and size of the magnets. Hence the blood is drawn to the area where magnets are placed thus increasing the blood circulation in the area. This in turn floods the affected area with oxygen and other nutrients in the blood. This then assists in healing the diseased area. Bottom line! Cancer cells cannot survive in oxygen rich environment. Read chapter on "The Amazing Oxygen Cure" in this book.

With this concept in mind magnets have been successfully used to treat cancer patients. Professor Goesta Wollin & Erika Enby had great success with use of magnets for curing different diseases including cancer.

One was the prolonged use of high gauss magnets to completely eliminate and control the pain of a man diagnosed with incurable liver cancer. Because of the use of strong North facing magnets applied over the site of pain, he was able to spend his last days with a minimum amount of discomfort without the use of morphine or any other deadening pain medication.

Two women, one with lung and another with breast cancer were able to minimize or completely eradicate any attendant pains in a similar way.

Finally, a man with a diagnosed brain tumor, fastened a strong neodymium magnet on a cap which he wore for half to one hour periods twice each day. He was reexamined after a period of several months and doctors were amazed to find that his tumor had shrunk.

Effect of Magnetic Fields on Tumor Growth and Viability

Readers who are research minded are advised to review this link from US National Library of Medicine and National Institute of Health.
https://www.ncbi.nlm.nih.gov/pmc/articles/PMC3155400/

Quick Summary: Our results showed that exposure of the mice to magnetic fields for 360 min daily for as long as 4 week suppressed tumor growth. Our study is unique in that it uses an in vivo imaging system to monitor the growth and progression of tumors in real time in individual mice. Our findings support further exploration of the potential of magnetic fields in cancer therapeutics, either as adjunct or primary therapy. An added potential advantage is that magnetic fields have the potential to cause less normal tissue damage, compared to more traditional treatments including Chemo and Radiation.

Magnetic nanoparticles to cure cancer

Please refer to this link from Medical News today:

http://www.medicalnewstoday.com/articles/270100.php

Quick summary: Scientists from Nanoprobes, Inc. claim that magnetic nanoparticles can cure cancer in just one treatment. Their findings are published in The international Journal of Nanomedicine. Dr. Hainfeld and Huang claim a success rate of 78-90% in mice. They are currently conducting more lab tests in preparation for FDA approval. Please do not miss this for valuable information.

Magnets that kill cancer cells

(Researchers devise a way to use magnets to make cells self-destruct)

Please review this link:
https://www.sciencenewsforstudents.org/article/magnets-kill-cancer-cells

Summary: Scientists at Yonsei University in South Korea developed the new technology. At once, cells started to die. After 24 hours of this magnetic therapy, more than half of the cancer cells were dead. It's too soon to know whether this magnetic therapy will be able to distinguish healthy cells from diseased cells! Hence further study is warranted.

Use of Flex Magnetic pads to treat cancer tumors.

Many experiments have shown reversal of cancer with use of Static Magnetic field. For example exposing the cancer cells with negative magnetic field using strong North Pole of a permanent magnet. Here is a simple way to achieve this with a use of flex magnetic pad as shown below.

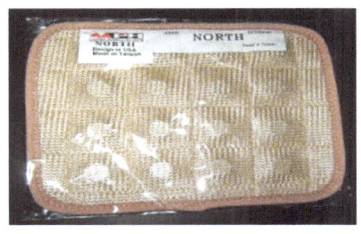

Available in USA at
http://www.healingwithmagnets.org/FLEX-MAGNETIC-PAD-WITH-16-MAGNETS-2500-Gauss-each-FLEX-MAG-16.htm

This flex Pad measures 5" x 6.5" and has 16 powerful magnets each 2500 gauss. All north is on one side and south on the other. These portable pads can be used standalone and can be easily inserted inside clothing touching the skin directly. Normally north side facing the skin. This way you can target specific body areas including abdominal and breast areas.

Simply insert it inside the clothing over the tumor area and hold it there in place with a surgical tape or clothing. Wear it all day/night when possible making sure the north side faces the tumor area. Remove it if you are being treated with Chemo therapy or radiation and during a bath. Also do not wear it if travelling by air or at airport security.

Note: Avoid use of magnetic therapy if you are pregnant or have any implants. Also stay away from close to heart area.

11. Intravenous Vitamin C Therapy

According to National Cancer Institute high dose Vitamin C has been studied as a treatment for patients with Cancer since the 1970s.

Laboratory studies have shown that high doses of vitamin C may slow the growth and spread
of prostate, pancreatic, liver, colon, and other types of cancer cells.

Some human studies of high-dose IV vitamin C in patients with cancer have shown improved quality of life, as well as improvements in physical, mental, and emotional functions, symptoms of fatigue, nausea and vomiting, pain, and appetite loss.

High-dose vitamin C may be given by intravenous (IV) infusion (through a vein into the bloodstream). When taken by intravenous infusion, vitamin C can reach much higher levels in the blood than when the same amount is taken by mouth. Studies have also shown that Vitamin C levels in the blood are higher when taken by IV than when taken by mouth, and last for more than 4 hours. Intravenous high-dose ascorbic acid has caused very few side effects in clinical trials.

- Combining high-dose vitamin C with certain types of chemotherapy may be more effective than chemotherapy alone:

- Ascorbic acid with arsenic trioxide may be more effective in ovarian cancer cells.
- Ascorbic acid with gemcitabine and epigallocatechin-3-gallate (EGCG) may be more effective in malignant mesothelioma cells.

- Another laboratory study suggested that combining high-dose vitamin C with radiation therapy killed more glioblastoma multiforme cells than radiation therapy alone.

However, not all laboratory studies combining vitamin C with anticancer therapies have shown benefit.

Combining dehydroascorbic acid, a particular form of vitamin C, with chemotherapy made it less effective in killing some kinds of cancer cells, while generally approved as a dietary supplement, the U.S. Food and Drug Administration (FDA) has not approved the use of IV high-dose vitamin C as a treatment for cancer or any other medical condition.

According to Dr. Frank Shallenberger, MD

Many if not most oncologists (cancer specialists) have the opinion that vitamins and other nutrients will decrease the effectiveness of chemo drugs.

In fact, the evidence is the opposite. Not only does the use of vitamins, especially antioxidant vitamins like vitamin C, not interfere with chemotherapy, it actually improves chemotherapy.

A recent study on the use of high-dose intravenous vitamin C with chemotherapy points this out.

The researchers took nine men and women with advanced (stage four) pancreatic cancer. They gave them all very high doses of intravenous vitamin C twice a week while at the same time giving them the chemotherapy drug gemcitabine. Then they measured the progression of the cancer, their quality of life, their blood chemistry values, and overall survival. Here's what happened.

According to the authors, side effects from the combination "were rare" and were limited to a few temporary cases of diarrhea and dry mouth. With a study as small as this, it's impossible to draw any clear conclusions about whether or not the combination worked better than the chemo drug alone.

But with that in mind, the average survival time of these patients was 13 (±2) months. Compare that to the average survival without the combination which is 5 (±1) months.

I think it's pretty clear that not only did the vitamin infusions not decrease the effectiveness of the chemotherapy, they probably enhanced it. In the researchers' own words, "Data suggest pharmacologic ascorbate [high-dose intravenous vitamin C] administered concurrently with gemcitabine is well tolerated. Initial data from this small sampling suggest some efficacy." For the past 12 years, I've been using a combination of ozone therapy, vitamin C therapy, and chemo in my advanced cancer patients. And every single time the results are significantly better than what would have happened with just the chemo. The patients not only live longer, their quality of life is much better.

Before you do any kind of conventional anti-cancer therapy — whether it's surgery, radiation, or chemotherapy — please find a doctor who is well versed in high-dose vitamin C, ozone therapy, nutrition, and detoxification to work with you while you're going through your treatments. And don't work with any Oncologist who has the audacity to say that you should quit all of your vitamins and other supplements because they are supposedly going to interfere with his treatments. The evidence is just not there.

To read all about DR. Shallenberger's credentials please visit

http://www.secondopinionnewsletter.com/Why-Dr-Frank.htm

12. Foods and Health Supplements

Did you know fasting kills cancer cells! Researchers have found that fasting reduces the side effects of chemotherapy and increases its effectiveness! Actually fasting makes chemo more toxic to cancer cells and it speeds up the destruction of tumors.

As a matter of fact research indicates that the fasting alone could soon replace chemotherapy!

So if you are fighting cancer now add fasting as part of your effective treatment.

There are few different types of fasts to consider.

1) Water fast: 80 ounces of water daily for up to 3 days. Do this if you are in overall good health.
2) Juice fast. 80 ounces of juice up to 5 days. Use fresh juice of carrots, apples, beets, celery and lemons. Also can use in addition wheatgrass and green juices.
3) Also consider intermittent fasting. For example alternate day fasting.
   Limit your intake to 500 calories one day, then eat normally next day.
   You can also fast for 16-18 hours every day. Just skip breakfast, eat lunch around noon, and dinner by 6 or 7 PM. Nothing after that.
   Just pick what works for you.

   Avoid breads, carbohydrates as they convert to glucose. Now you should know cancer cells feed on glucose and nothing but glucose!

So diet that includes meat, seafood, eggs, and non-starchy vegetables is fine but does not include breads, grains, rice, corn, pasta, and all sweets and fruits.

German researchers did exhaustive research of over 160 studies on diet and cancer, and concluded that restricting carbs prevents cancer and slows cancer growth.

Here is the summary of diet beneficial to you if you have cancer.

1. Avoid bread, pasta, sweets, soft drinks, and juices.
2. Use green leafy vegetables and high quality proteins like organic, grass fed beef, organic chicken and eggs, wild caught salmon and healthy fats including Olive oil, avocados and coconut oil.
3. Follow intermittent fasting. Consider 18 hour fast model as it seems to be a bit easy one.

Here is the list of Anti-Cancer foods

1. Cruciferous vegetables like Broccoli Sprouts. Eat raw or steamed half cup daily.
2. Cold water fish. Salmon, sardines and trout are rich in healthy omega-3 fats. Eat fish once or twice a week.

3. Tomatoes: Lycopene in tomatoes is effective in reducing the risk for prostate cancer. Consume cooked tomatoes several times a week.
4. Garlic. Allicin in garlic helps protect against cancers of colon, prostate, and kidneys. Consume garlic in all cooking.

5. Spinach. This green vegetable is ranked high for its ability to protect against cancer. Consume spinach daily cooked or in salads.
6. Turmeric: watch this video: https://youtu.be/4hoeYA4IGdc

Anti-Cancer Health Supplements:

1. Glutathione
It is one of the most powerful body's self-generated antioxidants.
It is also considered to be one of the most powerful anticancer agents manufactured by the body.
Glutathione works as a detoxification, or chelating, agent which works to remove heavy metals and other common toxins that our bodies are exposed to on a regular basis.
It is also used to aid in treatment of liver disease, ulcers and neurological conditions, as well as to assist in overall immune function. It is used by the liver to detoxify toxins including formaldehyde, acetaminophen, benzpyrene and many other compounds.

Glutathione levels decrease with age. Glutathione is involved in maintaining normal brain function. Therapeutically, Glutahione is used for several health conditions. Here are some worth noting.

Before radiation therapy

Liver disease including cirrhosis and fatty liver disease caused by alcohol: Clinical Research and Case studies show significant improvement in as little as 2 weeks.

Hematological conditions: myelofibrosis, acute leukemia, chronic myelocytic leukemia, lymphoma, polycythemia Vera.

Parkinson's disease, Alzheimer's disease, ALS (Lou Gehrig's disease).

Note: ORAL SUPPLEMENTATION OF ALL FORMS OF GLUTATHIONE DOES NOT RAISE TISSUE LEVELS OF GLUTATHIONE. Therefore the only way one could truly raise the reduced glutathione levels in body was by undergoing costly direct intravenous administration of reduced glutathione.

2. Green tea is likely the most healthful tea, and that's largely because of its unique, potent antioxidant, epigallocatechin gallate (EGCG). Drinking green tea can help protect against certain cancers, including bladder, breast, lung, stomach, pancreatic, and colorectal cancers.
   Studies show that drinking green tea might prevent atherosclerosis, improve cholesterol levels, and even reduce the risk of Parkinson's and Alzheimer's!

To take advantage of these benefits, make sure you're steeping your tea properly. You get the most antioxidant compounds in green tea when it is steeped for a long time—two hours—in cold water.

3. Apples: For example, phenolics, flavonoids and other chemicals found naturally in apples and other fruits and vegetables with "peels" can help fight breast cancer and kill other tumor cells. But you have to eat the peels. Apples in particular stood out among all fruit. A recent Finnish study reveals similar results.

You can now find a tremendous variety of apples even at your local grocery store. But it's best to wash those thoroughly to make sure there is no pesticide residue on the peel, which is that part you want to eat. Better yet– stick to organic apples.

4. Essiac Tea –A native herbal Cancer Remedy

5. The Top Super Foods That I Eat Every Day
By   Dr. Michael T Murray

https://youtu.be/mpP9Me1VVkU

These Cancer Causing Foods You Should Never Eat

1. Refined Sugar

2. Soda Pop

3. Processed meat

4. Red Meat (except grass-fed meat occasionally)

5. Microwave Popcorn

6. Regular fruit sprayed with Pesticides

7. Potato Chips

8. French Fries

9. Farmed Salmon

10. Canned Tomatoes. Use Organic
11. Hydrogenated Oils and trans fats White Flour and bread

12. Too much Alcohol

13. Pickles (Limit One large Pickle a day)

14. GMOs

15. Artificial Sweeteners

Attention Ladies!

A study recently presented at the American Association of Cancer Research found that women who eat large amounts of cabbage and other green cruciferous vegetables have far better breast health than women who forgo them.

Cruciferous vegetables include the cabbage family, such as red and white cabbage, Brussel sprouts and bok choy. Other types of vegetables in the cruciferous category include broccoli, cauliflower and leafy dark greens.

Not only do these nutrients fight existing cancer cells, but they also prevent cancer cells from forming in the first place.

Amazing Health Supplements You Need to Know About.

AHCC: The world's most researched specialty immune supplement supported by 20 human clinical studies, by over 30 papers published in PubMed-indexed journals and by more than 100 pre-clinical and in vitro studies.

Japan's leading alternative cancer therapy used in hundreds of cancer clinics throughout Asia.

Highly effective immuno-modulator used in over 700 clinics as a standard preventative regiment for all incoming patient to reduce the risk of hospital infections. The daily immune supplement of tens of thousands of healthy people in Japan and worldwide, seeking to help their bodies to fight the formation of abnormal cells, whose growth can lead to cancer, chronic disease and infections (such as the influenza / flu virus).

Learn more here: http://ahccresearch.com/

Also review this site regarding uses, side effects, interactions and dosing and more.

http://www.webmd.com/vitamins-supplements/ingredientmono-1110-AHCC.aspx?activeIngredientId=1110&activeIngredientName=AHCC

13. Resources

http://www.ncbi.nlm.nih.gov/pmc/articles/PMC351042
6/

https://www.youtube.com/watch?v=txmj5MXDN9A

https://www.youtube.com/watch?v=AOXuES4AUBw&
ebc=ANyPxKqrUqXk6aYOn62Q6zhIAJj6W2aXg3Rq
6G9D2PnaZBEMij_Xzw_0pRqu-
cFWxFLVfbR8EQCDCiEs749xhGrShpf__T84RA

http://www.webmd.com/cancer/

New Drugs to fight Cancer

The immunotherapy drugs they've created use our own immune system as a powerful and safe weapon against cancer, Alzheimer's and other diseases. These "checkpoint inhibitors" unleash the natural immune system, empowering T cells to attack tumors even harder than they normally do.

Immunotherapy drugs also help patients reduce their exposure to radical treatments such as chemotherapy or radiation.

These new drugs are proving effective. For instance, a study of nearly 5,000 advanced melanoma patients treated with Yervoy from Bristol-Myers Squibb found that 21% were still alive three years later. That's about 1,000 people who almost certainly would have died otherwise.

The Gaithersburg, Md.-based company Emergent BioSolutions Inc. (NYSE: EBS), has been producing a series of vaccines against key threats such as anthrax for more than a decade.

There company called Aptevo has been quietly amassing a deep portfolio of proven drugs now on the market, as well as a rich pipeline of treatments that are showing solid results in clinical testing. Based on its

innovative ADAPTIR immunotherapy technology, Aptevo has found the key to a range of new immunotherapy compounds targeting a broad range of treatments.

In recent years, many companies have been developing cancer-fighting drugs that use monoclonal antibodies, replicas of the body's natural immune cells. But these antibodies are not always effective and also come with a range of side effects. In contrast, ADAPTIR technology uses targeted proteins, which are more potent, have a shorter half-life and carry minimal side effects.

The approach has proven to be effective against cancers and blood disorders. This isn't just a science experiment. Aptevo is already selling four drugs based on ADAPTIR.

They target hemophilia; immune thrombocytopenic purpura (ITP), which causes excessive bleeding and bruising; shingles; and hepatitis B. Five more drugs are in clinical trials, targeting Alzheimer's, inflammatory bowel disease and several forms of cancer. As it spins off and has to pull its own weight, Aptevo intends to focus even more directly on **cancer vaccines** in coming years.Also check this site for additional information on Cancer Vaccines:

http://veritalife.com/cancer-vaccine-potential/

LATEST NEWS.

FDA Approves Pembrolizumab for Microsatellite Instability-High and Mismatch Repair Deficient Cancers.

See more at:

http://www.onclive.com/web-exclusives/fda-approves-pembrolizumab-for-microsatellite-instabilityhigh-and-mismatch-repair-deficient-cancers

Note: There is ton of information on this site.

Check my other books on Kindle.

1) HERBS FOR HEALTH AND HEALING (HEALTH SERIES Book 1) Kindle Edition
https://www.amazon.com/dp/B0080UVQUU

2) EDTA - THIS FOUR LETTER WORLD MAY SAVE YOUR LIFE: SUPPORTED BY ACTUAL CASE STUDIES (HEALTH SERIES Book 2)
https://www.amazon.com/dp/B00GHC88BI

3) HOW TO PREVENT AND REVERSE HEART DISEASES: and Even Avoid By-Pass (HEALTH SERIES Book 3) Kindle Edition
https://www.amazon.com/dp/B00B4CQ3GS

4) PAIN TREATMENT WITH MAGNETS (HEALTH SERIES Book 4) Kindle Edition
https://www.amazon.com/dp/B007IO7DN8

5) AMAZING GLUTATHIONE: Mother of All Anti-Oxidants to Live Longer and Healthy (HEALTH SERIES Book 5) Kindle Edition
https://www.amazon.com/dp/B00XWTX742

6) POWER OF CO-ENZYME Q 10: Health Supplement That Could Save Your Life (HEALTH SERIES Book 6) Kindle Edition
https://www.amazon.com/dp/B00ZRUBIZE